The Boogeyman in the Orange Bottle

A Love Story

as told by *TEAMS*

The Erick A Myrthil Story

ISBN: 978-0-692-10132-2
ISBN-13:

Prepared by Ebony Nicole Smith | Exclusively4Clergy | www.EbonyNicoleSmith.com

Edited by: CaTyra Polland, President of Polland Enterprises, LLC www.pollandllc.com

Cover Design by: Sarah Peck paintspeck@gmail.com

DEDICATION

This publication is dedicated to Elizabeth and to all those who have battled the prescription drug crisis this country has forgotten. For those who gave up when an outlet wasn't provided, you are not forgotten. I have been where you are and I'm making it my life's mission to win for all of us.

The Erick A Myrthil Story (TEAMS)

CONTENTS

Part 1: By the Numbers

Everyone has a boogeyman. Mine was in a bottle that cost
me a $1 per month

- TEAMS –

Since I was young child, I've never been afraid of horror
movies. Freddy, Chucky, and Jason were comical to
me. However, I began having regular nightmares in 2009. I
later discovered that this was caused by my prescription to
Aricept. I I was prescribed Aricept in 2008 to increase
brain activity. Shortly after I started taking Aricept I
noticed bad side effects. I did everything the doctor
ordered not knowing it would lead to dependency.

The prescription industry is a trillion dollar industry. Even
if you have not taken prescribed medications, someone you
know has. Many people can only function by taking
medication. Unfortunately, the side effects undoubtedly
outweigh the benefits.

For example, *Benzodiazepine (Benzos)* causes three-hundred deaths a day. *Benzos* treats anxiety. It has the fastest dependency rate of any prescribed medication. After forty-eight hours, your brain is becomes reliant on the narcotic. I was prescribed Benzodiazepine in the fall of 2010 as a last resort. I was also prescribed *Klonopin* to treat my insomnia. I wish I researched the drugs and its effects. I was not informed of how*Benzodiazepine* and *Klonopin* would change my brain's GABA (Gamma Aminobutyric Acid) censors. I was advised to continue taking them. I later traced my health problems to the prescription.

The prescriptions were helpful for the first ninety days. I felt like I could go out and fight crime. You would only understand if you know where I come from. I thought I had discovered a solution, I was wrong. The pharmaceutical industry has a job, which is to create customers not cures. I learned that the hard way.

The Numbers

Did you know that pharmaceutical corporations trade on Wall Street? Yes. Johnson & Johnson, the makers of many over the counter drugs including the very popular Aspirin, trade daily on the European market. Shameful because I believe 99% of their consumers are unaware. Did you know they produce Tylenol? I guarantee you have a bottle in your medicine cabinet as you're reading this. I researched the pharmaceutical industry, questioned how politics play a role in pharmaceuticals, currency and global trading with the dollar. The dollar copay costs you more than four quarters. It wreaks havoc on your health and can cost you your life.

The pandemic is maintained by the companies profiting from the pharmaceutical industry. We would be foolish to believe they are really working to change it, customers generate revenue after all. If you are cured, you are no longer revenue garnering to pharmaceutical companies. A long as your health insurance continues to pay for your visits and prescriptions you will be a consumer of their products. I have a great relationship with my doctor and I feel she truly does have my best interest at heart. However, I began questioning my wellbeing and sanity when I started taking my prescription.

Big pharmacy has America in a death grip and sadly, it's only getting tighter. To think that in a country of 323.1 million people the CDC (Center for Disease Control) has as many as 6 out of 10 adults taking at least one prescription (2016) is astonishing to say the least.

Furthermore, this alarming number is set to increase as the population grows. Plain and simple it's going to get a lot worse before it gets better. We condemn the guy selling drugs on the corner, while the drugs we obtain at our local pharmacy contain the same chemicals with similar side effects. The most egregious being death.

Pharmaceutical marketing cost is astronomical. At the expense of our day-to-day health, there is a goal to create lifelong dependent customers. The bottom line: dollars and cents.

The Numbers Don't Lie

A doctor's job is not to cure you anymore. It is to treat your condition. There is absolutely no money in the cure.

Even my friends and colleagues who work in the medical and pharmaceutical industry cannot deny that prescription is king. But even they couldn't deny that what's happening here should have us all in panic mode. We've become a prescription dependent people.

If the prescription addiction rates keep increasing at the pace they currently, will have a community of prescription drug addicts who are our family members, coworkers, friends, significant others and colleagues. This is certainly an epidemic. After force feeding us prescriptions for decades, we have a low tolerance for pain. Coupled with our high tolerance for numbness, we are in a dangerous place.

Part 2: Tale of Timmy

"Everyone has their own monsters. Mine lived in an
orange bottle that cost me $1 per month."

I awoke one morning feeling odd after my doctor
prescribed me a controlled substance to treat the
insomnia I had developed. After six months with no
improvement, I was prescribed a higher dosage. I became
dependent on the prescription.

Hello, all. I'm Timmy and this is my *boogeyman*.

It all started with a common pill to decrease my brain
digression. Around this time my insomnia worsened. I
didn't know this would push the snowball down the
mountain, it only gets worse from here.

I thought it was temporary, I followed the doctor's orders
when it appeared I'd grown immune to the 5mg dosage. I
complied when I was bumped to 10 mg per dosage. Your
brain stops responding to the dosage. The drug no longer

helps, you have become numb and need more of it or a different form to experience a change.

Why is it you have to be twenty-one to legally buy and consume alcohol but three year olds can take an antipsychotic medication? As much as we would like to assume this isn't a problem, it is. By labeling our children with newly developed ailments and prescribing medication we cause more damage. For example if you aren't talkative, you are evaluated and diagnosed with social anxiety. Rather than creating an action plan to improve the condition, your doctor prescribes a medication. I falsely believed my prescription did not have an impact on my being. I did not realize I developed a fear of doctors and hospitals due to the frequency of visits. I had become a pincushion for the many pills that followed. I wasn't sleeping, instead of addressing it I just adapted to being awake. I put full faith in the pharmaceutical industry.

"Take Two of These and Call Me in the Morning"

Pills are more of a hazard than a help. After over six years of being dependent on prescription drugs, I decided to quit cold turkey. It was the only logical answer to my insomnia. I had finally reached a point where enough was enough. In November 2016, I began to research narcotic withdrawal. Ironically, it was around the anniversary of being prescribed the *boogeyman*. I became frustrated with the doctors, nurses, and specialists. They only sought to put a band-aid over my issues. I became a guinea pig to test sleep medications.. The *band-aid* did nothing for the *boogeyman in the bottle*.

Fun with Prescription Drugs

I would love to say that the sleeping pills worked, solved my problems and life was great. Unfortunately, that was not the case. I was dependent on medication to sleep. Just as we condemn the guy selling drugs on the corner why don't we do the same to the pharmaceutical industry that prescribes much harsher drugs at little to no cost. Why do we accept this?

Cough syrup comes to mind when I think how many things are available to you without a prescription that if used incorrectly can have serious side effects. By using doctors as drug pushers, it's saddening to know that this country's prescription drug problem is partly it's own doing These trillion dollar monsters, aka *big pharma*, are major players on wall street in the housing market, and fortune 500 CEOs. The hardest fight of my thirty-one years was once I decided to stop taking the pills. This strengthened my reasons for writing this novel.

The flu vaccine is another pharmaceutical money maker. Everyone is encouraged to get the flu shot yearly to "help prevent" the infection. The vaccine actually has the flu virus in it along wither preservatives, formaldehyde, traces of aluminum and other chemicals. I encourage people to research what is being put into their bodies.

Another alarming pharmaceutical practice is the number of shots an infant must receive. The lethal injection that is administered to death row inmates is another cash cow.

HELP ME PLEASE!

Most of us have been to a doctor for something besides the common cold. We as a society have been conditioned to seek medical advice from trained specialists in the medical field. Within the last few decades the role of doctors have changed. Prescriptions and surgeries are more common than remedies. At one point my dentist prescribed me to high powered pain killers when she botched removing my wisdom tooth. This country is full of drug pushers and college educated drug dealers.

The Pain or the Hangover

Prescriptions are meant to eliminate or numb the pain. Unfortunately, this may lead to dependency. Prescription dosages are often increased when patient states the ailment is not improving. To avoid another change in dosage I began to drink heavily in addition to taking medication. I knew it was dangerous but it offered temporary, much desired relief.

I Need a Doctor

Doctors are pawns in the pharmaceutical industry. They are the lowest chamber of the cycle and the gateway to the product.

Julie B.

I met Julie Young around spring of 1998. She was the first Caucasian female I befriended. She used prescriptions for recreational highs. No one acknowledged that she was abusing her prescription. I witnessed the effects of the abuse firsthand. At the time I did not know that the human body responds to every substance it receives. I had yet to understand the long-term effects of taking prescribed medication.

Julie was prescribed Ritalin as a child. She began taking it for recreation to enjoy the high. To this day she currently uses drugs to function day-to-day. Julie was diagnosed with ADHD. ADHD is a formulated illness that was diagnosed for the first time in 1902. For Julie, the drug use would intensify as time passed. She would advance to harder drugs after the increase in milligrams was no longer effective. She eventually started using cocaine. She chased the high and numbing sensation. Although she would live a prosperous life, I wonder how different she would be *if* she was never introduced to prescription medication. In 1999 the total deaths of accidental drug overdoses was just over 4,000, That quadrupled over the last thirty years with the number estimated at almost 17,000. There is a large number of people taking prescriptions, not knowing it can lead to addiction, misery and chemical prescription drug dependency. Over four dozen Americans die daily from prescription drug overdoses.

The prestige of having the acronym MD behind your name is an admirable status. Although doctors are experts, they are not perfect. Prescriptions can be incorrect, ineffective and counterproductive.

A doctor's assessment is an educated guess. Although their intentions are good, diagnoses and prescriptions are not always accurate.

Timmy moved Rochester, NY from Detroit. Much like myself he developed a dependency and craved numbness.

Part 3: From the Horse's Mouth

They made me who I am and It must be known how.

~TEAMS~

I spoke with about nine people familiar with the pharmaceutical industry in preparation for this novel. The group included therapists, a doctor, a pharmacy technician, and two nurses one being an Registered Nurse and the other a nursing staff supervisor Certified Public Accountant.

While interviewing a physician I asked, "Are you aware how big of a crisis the prescription drug epidemic has become?" the physician answered, "It's like an iceberg what we see. What we know is the stuff above the surface. The bigger problem is rooted deep in our culture and fueled by the psychology of instant gratification, pain aversion, and often times an unrealistic expectation that the prescription will solve all the problems."

Another question I asked was if they were ever hesitant to prescribe medications. Surprisingly, they all replied yes. It showed me that they are pawns in the game of chess the pharmaceutical corporations are playing.

I was prescribed benzodiazepines to treat my chronic insomnia, it was everything I could have asked for. Ambien stopped working and the lack of sleep was showing in my day to day performance. The real problem was I was so drained of life I accepted and began the prescription. I laid down my sword, surrendered to the pharmaceutical industry's demands, and took the poison. In my research I learned about the damage these medications can do when taken for long periods of time. Pharmacists disclosed that many prescriptions to not rectify, correct or improve patient ailments, illnesses or conditions. Patients are merely victims of the trial and error method that has led to a rising number of annual deaths. In 2015 the number was approaching 200,000. The damage has been done and the problem is we cannot easily nor quickly reverse it.

Timmy's ordeal began with a painkiller prescription for an injury sustained from a work accident. He began to abuse the painkiller medication.

Timmy's Turmoil

Timmy moved to Rochester, NY to Detroit. Much like

myself he developed a dependence and craved numbness. Timmy inhaled deep while pumping gas, sniffed paint, drank hand sanitizer and used heroine. It was out of control until he was arrested for criminal trespassing while attempting to steal from a pharmacy delivery truck.

Timmy would spiral downward after he attempted robbery of the pharmacy truck. He was sentenced to two years and eight months for aggravated attempted strong-arm robbery. Just when it seemed Timmy had gotten his life together his tolerance for acetaminophen triggered a relapse. Timmy suffered a nearly fatal seizure due to heroin use.

Timmy was prescribed Vicodin to treat his chronic headaches. Unfortunately, he took the recommended dose on the bottle which slowed his breathing and his heart rate causing his death.

As a recovering addict I saw myself in Timmy so everything we spoke about applied to myself. I never looked down at him because we walked the same path. Truthfully, he inspired me to be better.

The Truth of the Stories

This tale of prescription and recreational drug use resonated with me. I was one of the lucky ones who kicked my habit with hard work and determination. I realized the fight was so much bigger than myself. The very citizens who mask their pain with pills, syrups, capsules, injections, therapies, and procedures suffer terrible and potentially fatal side effects.

Every single pill on the market has side effects. Many cases are greater than the original diagnoses they were prescribed to treat.

Part 4: Crisis in Our Cabinets

I Ain't Fraid of No Ghost

Think about everything we consume in life, how we react to that consumption and its chemicals Are prescriptions effective? Does it cure or improve the illness, impairment, ailment, disease or virus?

I am not a doctor, nurse, pharmacist, or medical industry expert. I am just an everyday guy whose life was turned upside down by taking pharmaceutical medications. After experiencing my own personal hell while going through a benzodiazepine withdrawal, I decided to address the issue.

Patients are customers who generate revenue. The pharmaceutical industry thrives on patient diagnosis and misery. The sad truth is that something is not done soon we'll be dealing with a future generations of prescription drug addicts. It is time to change the status quo.

The point of this book is in no way to get you to turn your back on medicine or your doctor. The reason I wrote this book is to get us, as a nation, to understand that we are not in a good position. The era of combating this problem needs to begin. There is no more time to waste.

The solution is our responsibility.

Let's put an end to the BOOGEYMAN IN THE ORANGE BOTTLE.

About TEAMS

TEAMS is an acronym that stands for *The Erick A Myrthil Story*. I first discovered my ability to write while being bedridden towards the end of 2014. I decided to write a memoir titled The Erick A Myrthil Story. *TEAMS* later became my pen name upon the release of the novel.

The day I decided to write about this travesty was during my withdrawal in the midst of my own misfortune. I made the decision that my second novel would be a narrative about benzodiazepines.

This novel tells my story as a prescription drug addict survivor. I wanted to tell my story to help others and highlight this epidemic. The greatest thing I have done in my life was kick my benzodiazepine dependence When I realized that those like myself had no resources, I made myself available as a case example and advocate.

If you or anyone you know is suffering from prescription drug dependency, please don't hesitate to call me 24/7 585-456-6109. I've been where you are. I believe you will get where I am.

Everyone is someone...don't ever forget that.

I am The Erick A Myrthil Story - *TEAMS*

www.ingramcontent.com/pod-product-compliance
Lightning Source LLC
Chambersburg PA
CBHW032301210326
41520CB00048B/5798